4/30/09 APPLE $21.95

CERVICAL CANCER

Current and Emerging Trends in Detection and Treatment

HEATHER HASAN

ROSEN
PUBLISHING®

New York

To my grandmother, Lee Francis, a cancer survivor

Published in 2009 by The Rosen Publishing Group, Inc.
29 East 21st Street, New York, NY 10010

First Edition

Library of Congress Cataloging-in-Publication Data

Hasan, Heather.
Cervical cancer: current and emerging trends in detection and treatment / Heather Hasan.
    p. cm.—(Cancer and modern science)
Includes bibliographical references and index.
ISBN-13: 978-1-4358-5007-1 (library binding)
1. Cervix uteri—Cancer—Popular works. I. Title.
RC280.U8H375 2009
616.99'466—dc22

                                      2008019938

Manufactured in the United States of America

On the cover: Colored scanning electron microscope image of HeLa cervical cancer cells. The cells have just replicated and are still connected by a cytoplasmic bridge.

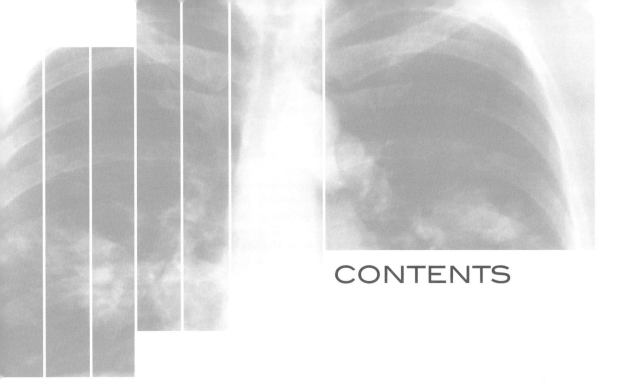

CONTENTS

INTRODUCTION

Eva Perón was born into poverty in 1919 in a small town in Argentina. She was the daughter of a nobleman and his mistress. Because her father never acknowledged her as his daughter, she was very poor. At the age of fifteen, Eva made her way to Argentina's capital, Buenos Aires. There, she followed her dream of becoming an actress. She became a singer, and, because of her talent and personality, soon rose to the top of her profession. In 1944, Eva met her future husband, Juan Perón. They were married the following year. In 1946, Juan Perón was elected president of Argentina, and Eva became the First Lady.

Though her husband was a ruthless dictator, Eva was dearly loved by the poor and working-class people of Argentina. She became affectionately known as Evita, meaning "little Eva." Evita quickly became the most popular person in Argentina. She was powerful within the trade unions that spoke on behalf of the labor rights of working-class citizens. She also founded the Eva Perón Foundation, a charitable organization that helped the poor. Through the foundation, Evita

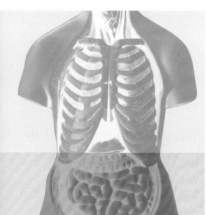
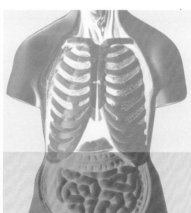
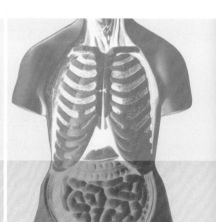

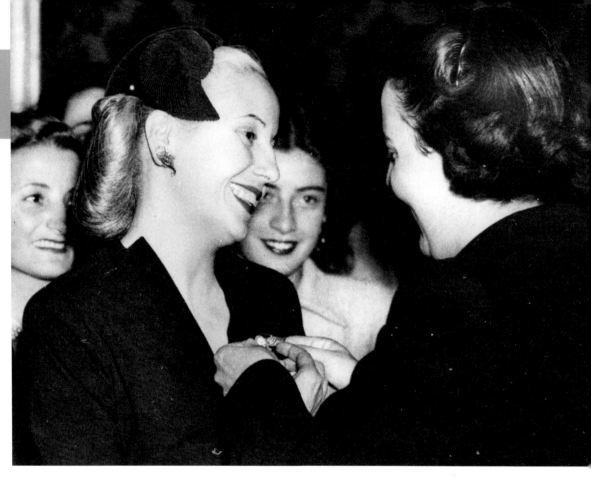

Eva Perón is presented with an insignia by the Institute for Work of Argentina in 1950. Perón was widely adored for her good deeds done on behalf of the working class and poor of Argentina.

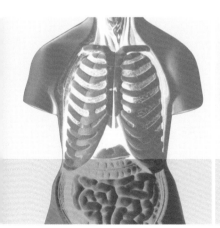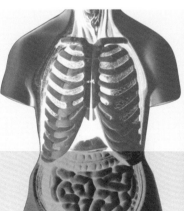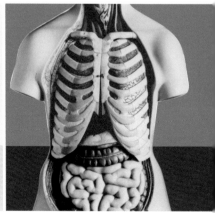

employed thousands of workers. Each year, the organization distributed many sewing machines, shoes, and cooking pots to needy people. Under Evita's leadership, the organization also built new houses, hospitals, schools, and orphanages. Evita also founded Argentina's first large female political party, called the Female Perónist Party.

In 1950, at the age of thirty, Evita fainted in public. She was diagnosed with inflammation of the appendix. Her doctors removed her appendix, but Evita never really recovered. She continued to be weak and tired. Then, Evita began to have terrible vaginal bleeding. An Argentinean doctor diagnosed her with cervical cancer. However, her husband, Juan Perón, never told her of the diagnosis. In 1951, Evita was operated on by a famous American cancer surgeon, George T. Pack. Dr. Pack tried to remove the large amount of cancer inside her, but the cancer had already spread. When she awoke, Evita was told that the surgery was a success. She still was not told that she had cancer. Soon after that, at the age of thirty-three, Evita died from cervical cancer. It is interesting to note that Perón's first wife had also died of cervical cancer.

This book is about the relationship between modern science and cervical cancer, so it focuses quite a bit on technology and medical advances. But the most important message to take away is that cervical cancer is basically a sexually transmitted disease (STD) caused by the human papillomavirus (HPV). This knowledge alone allows us to do a lot to prevent cervical cancer. Among the most important things to be informed about are healthy sexual behavior, use of preventative medicines, and early detection of abnormal cells with routine gynecologic care.

Shortly before her death, Evita was given the official title of "Spiritual Leader of the Nation." She had also expressed a desire to run for vice president. Who knows what she may have accomplished if she had survived? Unfortunately for her, she did not have the benefits of today's scientific knowledge and technology. A woman in her place now would most likely survive her fight against cervical cancer. However, both Evita and her doctors did not have the knowledge that we have today. Cervical cancer is still one of the leading causes of death in women, but women and their doctors are much better informed. This book will help you, too, to be better informed about the causes, diagnosis, staging, and treatment of cervical cancer.

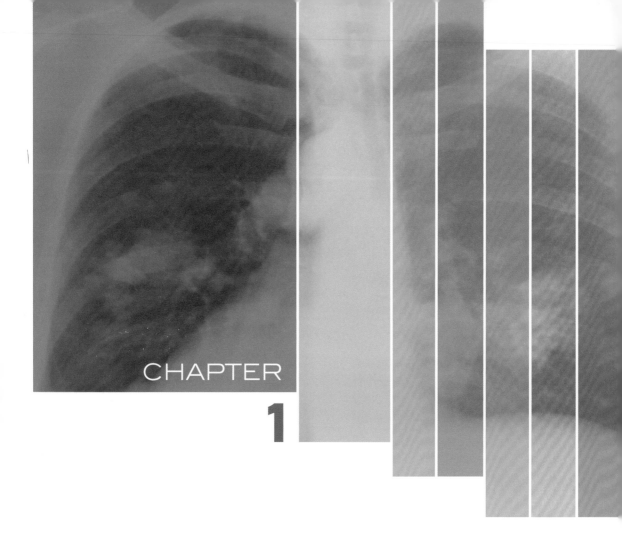

WHAT IS CERVICAL CANCER?

The human body is made up of billions of cells. Cells are the smallest units of living things. They are so small that they can only be seen with a microscope. Cells are the building blocks of life. Different cells group together to form the tissues and organs of the body. Normal, healthy cells grow and multiply to form new cells. However, some cells in the body are not normal.

Cancer cells are abnormal or damaged cells. Normal body cells repair themselves or die when they are damaged. However, cancer cells are able to multiply to form more abnormal cells. Normal, healthy cells divide in a planned way, but cancer cells reproduce without order. The cancerous cells form excess tissue called a tumor. Cervical cancer occurs when abnormal cells grow on the cervix, a part of the female reproductive system.

THE REPRODUCTIVE SYSTEM

The female reproductive system allows a woman to produce eggs, have sexual intercourse, protect and nourish a baby until it is fully developed, and give birth. A female's internal reproductive organs include the vagina, uterus, fallopian tubes, and ovaries. The vagina is a muscular tube that goes from the vaginal opening to the uterus. The uterus, or womb, is shaped like an upside-down pear. It houses a fetus until the fetus is ready to be born. The muscles of the uterus then help to push the baby out.

The two fallopian tubes attach to the uterus. These tubes are about as wide as a piece of spaghetti. The fallopian tubes flare open at the ovaries, which are the organs that produce, store, and release eggs. (*Ova* is Latin for "eggs.") The ovaries are about the size and shape of unshelled almonds. Once an egg is released from an ovary, it travels into the fimbria, which is the fringed, open end of the fallopian tubes. From there, numerous tiny, hair-like cilia in the lining of the fallopian tube sweep the egg toward the uterus.

The cervix is the name for the lowest part of the uterus. The word "cervix" comes from the Latin word for "neck." The cervix connects the uterus with the vagina, or birth canal. The cervix is a passageway with strong, thick walls. The opening of the cervix is very narrow, but it is able to expand. During menstruation, the cervix stretches slightly to allow the lining of the uterus to be released. It is this stretching—along with the contracting of the uterus—that is thought to cause menstrual cramping. During childbirth, the cervix is able to expand up to 3.9 inches (10 centimeters) to let the baby out. The cervix is made

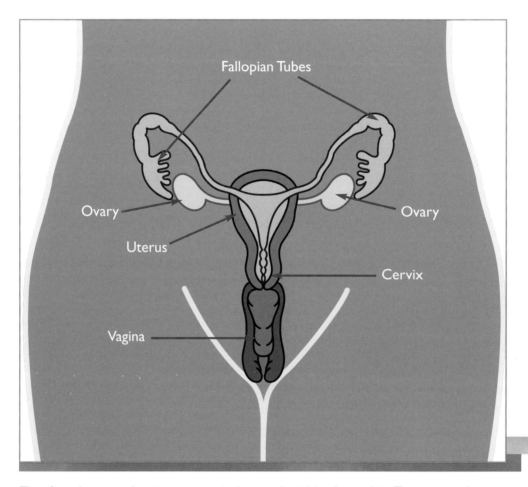

The female reproductive system is located within the pelvis. The internal reproductive organs include the vagina, the ovaries, the fallopian tubes, and the uterus. The cervix connects the lowest part of the uterus to the vagina.

of connective tissue, a binding or supportive tissue. It is lined with a mucous membrane, a moist lining that covers and protects it. The mucous membrane found in the cervix is similar to the mucous membrane that lines the mouth.

TYPES OF TUMORS

In some cases, tumors are benign, or noncancerous. These tumors do not grow in an unlimited, aggressive manner, and they do not invade surrounding tissues. Most of these benign tumors are harmless to the health of the person. They can usually be removed, and they do not grow back. Two types of benign tumors are fibromas and adenomas.

Malignant tumor cells, on the other hand, invade and destroy nearby, healthy tissues. Unlike benign tumor cells, they are also able to travel through the lymph and blood vessels to other parts of the body. Lymph is a colorless body fluid that contains white blood cells. Lymph vessels transport lymph throughout the body in much the same way that blood

AN EARLY RECORD OF CANCER

Cancer was named by the Greek physician Hippocrates. He called it *karkinos*, a word that was used to describe a crab. Hippocrates thought cancer looked like a crab. Cancer was known long before Hippocrates named it, however. The oldest written record of cancer appears on an Egyptian papyrus dating to 1500 BCE. (Papyrus is an ancient form of writing paper.) The document described eight cases of breast cancer. The Egyptians attempted to treat this cancer with a hot instrument they called "the fire drill." There was evidence that the Egyptians understood the difference between malignant and benign tumors. Ancient Egyptians also described the surgical removal of cancers on the skin's surface. They did this in a way that is similar to how we do it today.

This illustration shows the female lymphatic system. Lymph vessels transport lymph fluid, which is rich in immune cells that fight infection. Unfortunately, the lymphatic system also gives malignant cervical cancer cells a means to circulate to other organs.

vessels transport blood. After traveling through the body, malignant cancer cells start new tumors in other areas of the body. This process is called metastasis. When a cancer spreads in this way, it is said to have metastasized. Death occurs from cancer when the spreading of the cancer cannot be stopped. The cancerous cells take the place of healthy cells and multiply. This causes organ systems to fail, and the body cannot properly function.

Tumor cells may spread to other parts of the body, but the type of cancer is the same as the original growth. In other words, if cancer were to spread from the cervix to the lungs, it would still be considered cervical cancer. When it spreads, cervical cancer most often spreads to the intestines, bladder, lungs, and liver.

TYPES OF CERVICAL CANCER

The names of the different types of cancer cells can be very confusing. Cancers are named for the areas in which they develop. Cervical cancer, for example, begins in the lining of the cervix. The surface of the cervix contains two different types of cells: columnar epithelial cells and squamous epithelial cells. Epithelial cells are the cells that cover the body surfaces. Columnar epithelial cells and squamous epithelial cells appear different under a microscope. The columnar epithelial cells are tall and packed tightly next to one another. Squamous cells are thin, flat, and long, and they pile up on one another.

Cancers are put in categories according to the cells from which they originally formed. Cervical cancer that develops from squamous epithelial cells is called squamous cell carcinoma. Cervical cancer that develops from columnar epithelial cells is called adenocarcinoma. Most cervical cancers are squamous cell carcinomas. Squamous cell carcinoma is responsible for about 80 to 90 percent of all cervical cancers. The tumors of squamous cell carcinoma look like small lumps or ulcers of different sizes.

Adenocarcinoma is the second most common form of cervical cancer. Adenocarcinoma originates from columnar epithelial cells, the cells that make up the glands in the cervix. The glands of the cervix excrete mucus. About 10 to 20 percent of cervical cancers are adenocarcinomas. There are four types of cervical adenocarcinoma: clear cell adenocarcinoma, papillary adenocarcinoma, mucinous adenocarcinoma, and adenosquamous carcinoma.

Clear cell adenocarcinoma is fairly rare. The tumors look like polyps, or abnormal growths of tissue. Papillary adenocarcinoma is a rare but recognized form of cervical adenocarcinoma. It is found in young women, including teenagers. Mucinous adenocarcinoma is seen under the microscope as cells surrounded by pools of mucus.

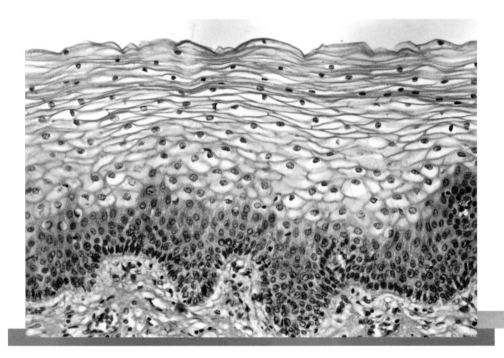

Squamous cells, like those shown here, are thin, flat, and long. They stack up on top of one another. The word "squamous" comes from the Latin word squama, *meaning "the scale of a fish or serpent," which these cells resemble.*

Scientists think that mucus allows cancer cells to spread faster. Therefore, mucinous carcinomas are considered to be more aggressive and harder to treat. Adenosquamous carcinoma has characteristics of both squamous cell carcinomas and adenocarcinomas. Unfortunately, adenosquamous carcinoma tumors grow very fast. Cervical adenocarcinoma is most common in women over the age of forty-five, but it can occur at any age, even during the teenage years.

Adenocarcinomas are becoming more common in women who were born in the last thirty years, though no one knows exactly why.

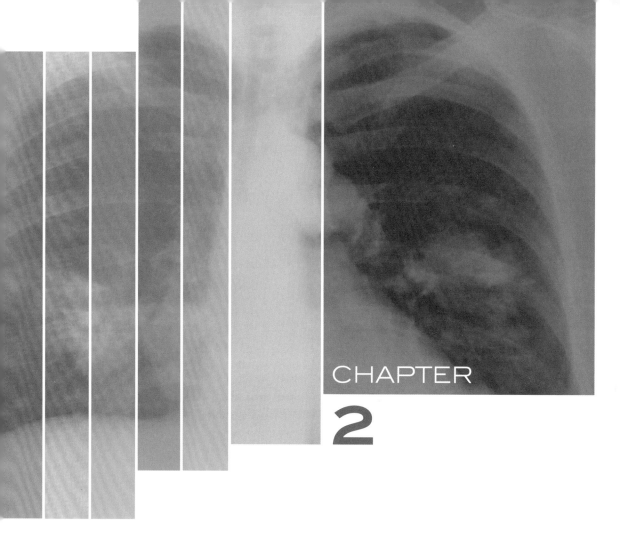

CHAPTER

2

WHO IS AT RISK?

Around the world, there are about five hundred thousand new cases of cervical cancer each year. About 80 percent of these cases occur in women who are living in developing countries. Cervical cancer can usually be prevented by early detection of cell changes, but medical treatment in developing countries is not as advanced as it is in North America or Europe. In developing countries, cervical cancer is the second most common cause of cancer death for women. In contrast, cervical cancer is only the fourteenth most common cause of cancer death for women in the United States.

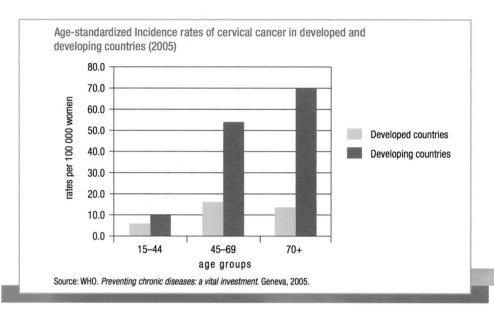

Age-standardized Incidence rates of cervical cancer in developed and developing countries (2005)

Source: WHO. *Preventing chronic diseases: a vital investment.* Geneva, 2005.

This bar graph shows the rates at which women in different age groups develop cervical cancer. Clearly, after age forty-five, women in developing countries (represented by the darker-colored bars) are at a much greater risk than women in developed countries (lighter-colored bars).

It is clear that the vast majority of cervical cancers are caused by infection with the human papillomavirus. There are about one hundred different strains, or types, of HPV. Of these, about thirty different strains are considered to be sexually transmitted diseases. Several risk factors for cervical cancer are well documented, yet no one knows for sure why some people infected with HPV get cancer and others don't. HPV is a very common infection among the U.S. general public. About four out of every five sexually active people, both men and women, are infected with HPV at some point. However, only about one in four American women tests HPV-positive with the strains that can develop into cervical cancer.

SEXUALLY TRANSMITTED DISEASES

Sexually transmitted diseases are infections that can be transferred from one person to another through sexual contact. Some examples of STDs include human immunodeficiency virus (HIV), gonorrhea, herpes, chlamydia, and HPV. According to the Centers for Disease Control and Prevention (CDC), more than fifteen million new cases of sexually transmitted diseases are reported each year in the United States. Young people between the ages of fifteen and twenty-four are at the greatest risk for getting an STD.

The best way to prevent getting an STD is to practice abstinence. When people practice abstinence, they avoid any kind of sexual activity. Condoms are useful for preventing some sexually transmitted diseases, like HIV and gonorrhea. However, they are less effective at protecting people from getting herpes and chlamydia. Condoms offer very little protection against HPV, the leading cause of cervical cancer. This is because HPV is transmitted through skin contact, and a condom does not cover all of the skin that comes into contact during sexual intercourse. Most STDs are treatable. Some, however, are becoming resistant to traditional antibiotics. (Gonorrhea is an example.) This means that the antibiotics have little or no effect on the disease. Other STDs, like herpes and acquired immunodeficiency syndrome (AIDS), have no cure. A cure has not yet been found for HPV infection either.

Getting infected with sexually transmitted diseases—chlamydia and HIV especially—is a risk factor for developing cervical cancer. Therefore, women who have had multiple sex partners are at a higher risk for cervical cancer. Women who begin having sexual intercourse at an earlier age also appear to be at a greater risk for developing cervical cancer. This may be because immature cells in the cervix of young women are more fragile and likely to be damaged by intercourse.

CAN HPV CAUSE CANCER IN MEN?

Many strains of HPV can infect both men and women. Men do not have cervixes, but HPV can still cause cancer in men. Cancers of the penis and anus in men are strongly linked to HPV. Men can be infected with HPV during sexual intercourse through small cuts on their penises or anuses. However, both penile and anal cancers are very rare. They also have very high cure rates when they are diagnosed early.

CERVICAL CANCER AND THE HUMAN PAPILLOMAVIRUS

HPV is a virus. Viruses are not living things, but they use living things to reproduce. Viruses are basically genetic material—deoxyribonucleic acid (DNA) or ribonucleic acid (RNA)—inside a protein capsule. They inject their genetic material into a living cell. Then, the virus DNA takes over the cell's machinery to make copies of itself. When enough new viruses have been produced, the cell bursts, releasing them. These viruses, in turn, attack other cells, leading to infection. Viruses are microscopic. In fact, a speck of dust is ten thousand times bigger than an HPV particle. Despite their size, however, viruses are responsible for many human illnesses, from the common cold to AIDS.

HPV mainly infects skin, or epithelial cells. The virus is transmitted between two people by direct skin contact. Depending on the type of HPV, an infected person may or may not experience symptoms. HPV is separated into two categories: low-risk HPV and high-risk HPV. A person infected with a low-risk HPV will usually develop genital warts.

These look like miniature, skin-colored cauliflower florets. Genital warts usually develop a few weeks to a few months after exposure, but sometimes it takes years for the warts to appear. Aside from genital warts, most people infected with low-risk HPV experience no other complications.

Women infected with high-risk HPV experience few or no symptoms. This means that people can get infected with HPV and pass it on without even knowing that they have it. However, women with high-risk HPV are at a significantly greater risk for developing cervical cancer. It is no coincidence that both Evita Perón and Juan Perón's first wife died

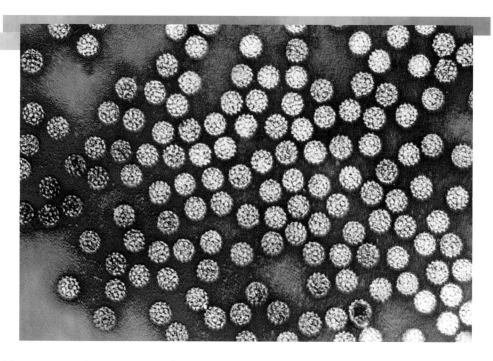

Human papillomaviruses, shown here, contain just two strands of DNA inside a round shell, or envelope. They resemble golf balls when viewed with an electron microscope.

of cervical cancer. (See the Introduction on page 4.) It is likely that these three people shared the same HPV virus.

It is important to note that a person can be infected with more than one strain of HPV at the same time. The strain of HPV that causes genital warts is not likely to lead to cervical cancer. However, someone with genital warts may also have a strain of HPV that does.

HPV infection is linked to almost all cervical cancer (99.7 percent). Being infected with HPV, therefore, is the major risk factor for developing cervical cancer. However, just because a woman is infected with HPV does not necessarily mean that she will develop cervical cancer. Many times, a woman's body can fight off the virus on its own. In fact, of the millions of cases of women with HPV infection, only about 0.2 percent progress to cancer. Cervical cancer is usually detected in middle-aged women. However, most of these women would have been infected with the HPV strain that caused their cancer while they were still in their teens and twenties. It may take as long as ten to twenty years for the

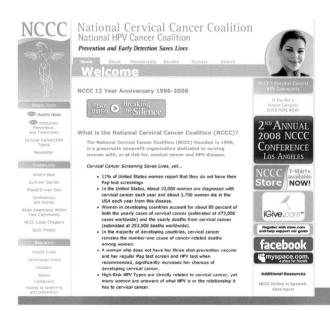

Here is the home page of the National Cervical Cancer Coalition (www.nccc-online.org). This organization, which was founded in 1996, is dedicated to informing women about cervical cancer and HPV.

cancer to develop. Therefore, it is important for teenage girls to be aware of the risks of HPV.

OTHER RISK FACTORS FOR CERVICAL CANCER

Infection with HPV is the most important factor in the development of cervical cancer. However, the physical conditions and behaviors listed below may also increase a woman's chances of developing cervical cancer.

SMOKING

Smoking cigarettes is considered a key risk factor for cervical cancer. Smokers are at least twice as likely to develop cervical cancer as non-

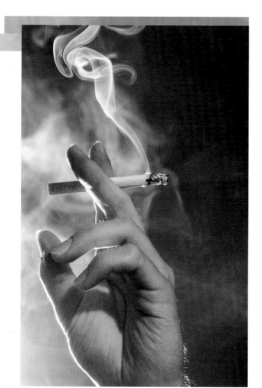

smokers. Smoking is known to suppress the body's immune system. This means when a person smokes, it is harder for his or her body to fight off infections, including HPV infection. Also, when a person smokes, the chemical nicotine is absorbed through the lungs. The nicotine is transported throughout the person's body by the blood-stream. Nicotine can be broken

Smoking cigarettes is a risk factor for developing not only cervical cancer but also many other kinds of diseases.

down into cancer-causing chemicals. Some of these cancer-causing chemicals have been found in the cervical mucous of women who smoke. The risk for developing cervical cancer seems to increase with the amount of cigarettes a woman smokes and the number of years she has been smoking.

IMMUNE SYSTEM

Women who have had many pregnancies also tend to be at a greater risk for developing cervical cancer. The exact reason for this is unclear. However, it may be due to the fact that a woman's immune system is suppressed during pregnancy. This means it is harder for a pregnant woman to fight off infections. Going through this multiple times may make a woman more vulnerable to HPV infection. Cervical cancer is also seen more often in other cases where a woman's immune system is weaker. For example, a woman infected with HIV has a weakened immune system, so it is more difficult for her body to fight off HPV infection. This puts her at a greater risk for developing cervical cancer.

DIET AND NUTRITION

Poor nutrition and a lack of exercise put a woman at a greater risk for developing cervical cancer. Studies show that cancer rates, in general, are lower among people who exercise regularly and eat plenty of fruits and vegetables. Exercise and a healthy diet help to control obesity. There is a strong connection between obesity and cancer. The death rate among women with cervical cancer is higher among those who are obese.

AGE

A woman's age is also a factor. The risk of cervical cancer rises with age. Women can be diagnosed with cervical cancer as early as their teens. However, the risk of developing cervical cancer begins increasing after the age of twenty-five.

HEALTH CARE

A woman's socioeconomic status is a risk factor for cervical cancer. Women who have lower incomes or who are economically disadvantaged tend to have limited access to medical care. In the United States, an African American woman is twice as likely to die from cervical cancer

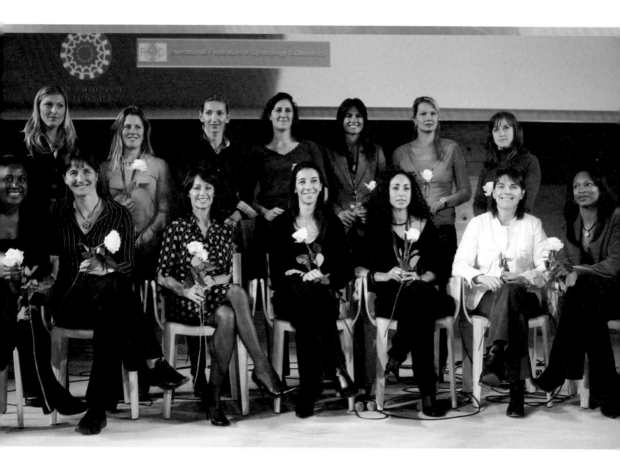

Several high-profile women were invited to attend the First Global Summit on Cervical Cancer in Paris in March 2007. Their fame helped raise global awareness about the importance of good health care with regard to cervical cancer prevention.

as is a Caucasian woman. The death rate among Hispanic and Native American women from cervical cancer is also higher. The increased death rate among these groups is most likely related to poor health care. When a woman does not have adequate health care, her cervical cancer may not be discovered until it is too late. As mentioned before, the death rate in developing countries is even higher than those in the United States. The highest occurrence of cervical cancer in the world is in sub-Saharan Africa and South America. Many women in these regions lack access to quality preventative health care.

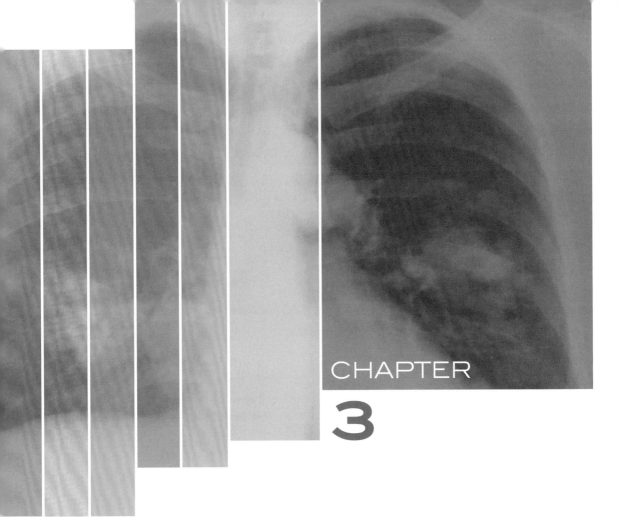

DIAGNOSING CERVICAL CANCER

Cervical cancer does not usually have any symptoms in the early stages. As the disease progresses, however, there are some signs to watch out for. One of the most common symptoms in later stages is abnormal vaginal bleeding. Abnormal vaginal bleeding includes bleeding after sexual intercourse, in between periods, heavier or longer-lasting menstrual bleeding, or bleeding after menopause. (Menopause is the time in a woman's life when she stops menstruating, usually occurring around the age of fifty.) Another common symptom is pain during or after sex. In advanced stages, cervical cancer causes pain in the back, the pelvic area, and the legs. Other symptoms include blood in the urine, as well as pain while urinating. Once symptoms such as pain and bloody urine are detected, it is often too late for effective therapy. However, these symptoms usually have other causes and are not indicative of cervical cancer. Whatever the root cause, it is important for women to see their doctors right away.

VISITING THE GYNECOLOGIST

A gynecologist is a doctor who specializes in the health of the female reproductive system. This includes the diagnosis and treatment of disorders and diseases. Any woman who is sexually active or is over the age of eighteen should see a gynecologist regularly. Getting routine gynecology care will help a young woman to understand how her body functions. A gynecologist will ask the woman questions and address any concerns that she has. Visiting the gynecologist can help a young woman to understand the reproductive cycle and establish what is normal for her.

Routine gynecological care will also help teenagers understand why it is healthier for them to refrain from sexual activity until they are older. It can also help them learn how to protect themselves from sexually transmitted diseases if they do decide to become sexually active. It is important to see a gynecologist regularly so that any problems can be identified and treated before they get worse.

During an annual visit, a gynecologist will visually check a woman's vaginal walls and cervix for signs of infection or disease. Some things to look for are wounds, redness, swelling, or unusual discharge. The gynecologist will feel the uterus and the ovaries to make sure they are a normal size. (A swollen uterus could indicate a problem.) The gynecologist will also do a breast exam to look for signs of breast cancer. Finally, the gynecologist will collect a sample of cervical cells using a plastic or wooden spatula or brush. This part of the exam is called the Pap smear.

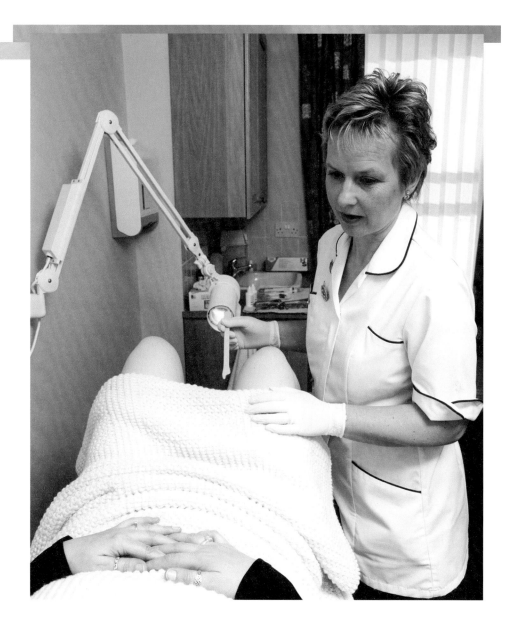

Gynecologists are on the front lines when it comes to helping women maintain good sexual health. Here, a gynecologist prepares a patient for a Pap smear.

THE PAP SMEAR

The Pap smear is one of the most important cervical cancer screening tests available. "Pap" is short for Papanicolaou, the last name of the inventor of the test. George Papanicolaou invented the Pap smear in the 1940s. The test is used to identify abnormal cervical cells before they become life threatening. Prior to the invention of the Pap smear, cervical cancer killed more women in the United States than any other form of cancer. Since the Pap smear has become a regular preventative screening test, the number of U.S. women developing cervical cancer has dropped by 75 percent. Today, getting the Pap smear is one of the most important things a woman can do to prevent dying from cervical cancer.

GEORGE PAPANICOLAOU

George Papanicolaou was born in 1883 in Greece on the island of Evia. As a boy, he loved the sea and longed to join the navy. However, he decided to follow in his father's footsteps and study medicine. Papanicolaou studied at the University of Athens, graduating with honors. In 1910, he dedicated his life to biological research. He moved to New York, and, in 1914, he took a job at the Pathological Anatomical Laboratory of the New York Hospital. Papanicolaou worked for almost fifty years without taking a holiday. It is said that he gave his life away for the women of the world. In fact, the invention of the Pap smear has saved countless lives since its invention in the 1940s. Papanicolaou's goal in life was not to become rich but to do something worthy of a good human being. He definitely accomplished that goal!

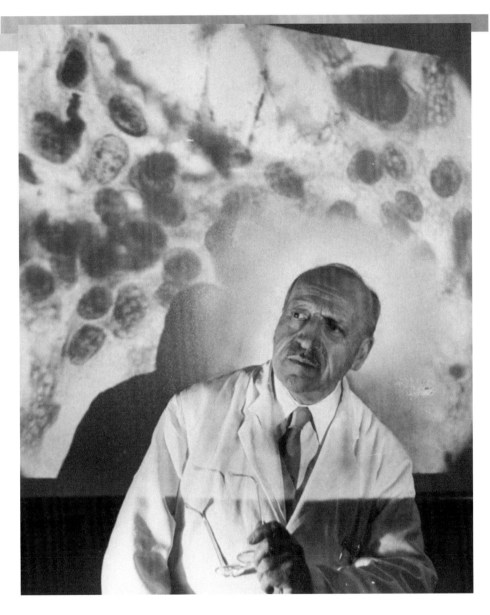

George Papanicolaou is shown here in front of a slide of cancer cells. As the inventor of the Pap smear, Papanicolaou has helped save the lives of countless women.

First, the gynecologist collects a sample of cervical cells. These are put in a jar with a Pap fixative, an alcohol-based liquid that preserves and protects the cells. The sample is sent to a laboratory, where a cyto-pathologist examines the cells under a microscope. A cytopathologist is someone who is trained to recognize abnormalities in cells. A cell contains two main parts: a nucleus, which contains the genetic material, and the cytoplasm, which is the watery substance inside the cell. Under a microscope, the nucleus of a normal cell appears as a small, dark, dense structure near the center of the cell. A large amount of a normal cell is made up of cytoplasm. In an abnormal cell, the nucleus is irregular and unusually large. An abnormal cell also contains very little cytoplasm. The presence of abnormal cervical cells is a warning sign for cancer.

If abnormal cells are identified early on, then steps can be taken that may prevent the onset of cervical cancer. Therefore, health care

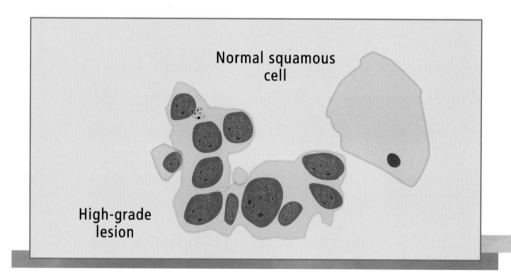

This illustration shows the structural difference between abnormal squamous cells in a high-grade lesion (left) and a normal squamous cell (right). High-grade lesions may progress into cervical cancer.

professionals recommend that women begin having yearly Pap smears when they become sexually active or when they reach the age of eighteen. The major reason that women develop cervical cancer is that they are not getting regular Pap smears that could have detected cell changes before they became cervical cancer. Most women who are diagnosed with cervical cancer have not had a Pap smear in five or more years.

ABNORMAL PAP RESULTS

If the results of a Pap smear are abnormal, then there are other tests that can determine the problem. As many as 20 percent of Pap smears are inaccurate. This means that the results seem abnormal when they aren't. Sometimes, for example, abnormal results are due to inflammation or infections such as yeast infections. These can cause the cells to look atypical under a microscope, though the cells might turn out not to be dangerous after all. Infections can usually be treated with antibiotics. After the infection has been treated, the Pap smear can be repeated. A second Pap test usually shows whether the first test results were correct.

If repeat Pap tests are not normal, or a woman tests positive for HPV, then a gynecologist will recommend that she undergo a colposcopy. This procedure takes about ten to fifteen minutes and can be done right in the gynecologist's office. For this procedure, the gynecologist uses a colposcope, which is an instrument that illuminates and magnifies the cervix. The doctor can then take a biopsy sample from the suspicious area. The sample obtained in a biopsy is larger than what is scraped off the cervix during a Pap smear, so the results are more accurate. A pathologist examines the tissue sample under a microscope. Pathologists are scientists who specialize in disease. The results of a biopsy reveal whether or not a woman has cervical cancer. The results can help the doctor determine if there are potentially dangerous pre-cancerous cells that need to be removed.

MYTHS AND FACTS

MYTH I am too young to worry about cervical cancer.

FACT Ovarian cancer has the highest death rate of any reproductive system cancer in women.

MYTH If a woman has HPV, she will develop cervical cancer.

FACT HPV infection is very common in the United States, and it is linked to almost all cases of cervical cancer. However, only about one-fifth of 1 percent of the millions of women who have HPV will develop cervical cancer. In most cases, the virus goes away on its own without causing any problems.

MYTH If a woman is diagnosed with cervical cancer, she is going to die from it soon.

FACT More than 95 percent of the women treated at the earliest stage of cervical cancer (stage 1) survive at least five years after treatment. Survival rates go down as the disease is detected in later stages.

MYTH If a woman has an abnormal Pap smear, it means she has cervical cancer.

FACT Pap smears are not perfect, and their results are occasionally inaccurate. Sometimes, an infection can cause cervical cells to look different under the microscope. If the results of a Pap smear are abnormal, there are more accurate follow-up tests that can tell whether a patient has cervical cancer.

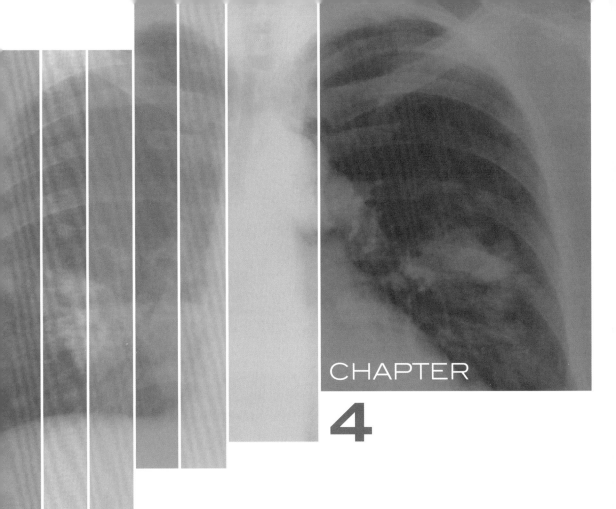

THE STAGES OF CERVICAL CANCER

Cervical cancer usually develops slowly. At the beginning, healthy cells in the cervix begin to develop abnormally. The abnormal cells can then become cancerous. Once a diagnosis of cancer is determined with a biopsy, doctors try to figure out how far the cancer has spread. This process is known as staging. Cervical cancer staging describes the size of the tumor on the cervix, how deeply the tumor has invaded the tissues within and around the cervix, and if the cancer has spread to the lymph nodes or other organs (metastasis). Staging is an important process because doctors use it to come up with a treatment plan. Different stages of cervical cancer need to be treated differently in order to obtain the best results.

Doctors must do a thorough examination in order to properly stage cervical cancer. This may include chest X-rays and a computed tomography (CT) scan to see if the cancer has spread throughout the body. It could also include ultrasound and magnetic resonance imaging (MRI) tests, which are used to look at things such as bones, the liver, lymph nodes, and the spleen. A doctor might also suggest a protosigmoi-doscopy. This test uses a lighted scope to examine the rectum and colon. All of these tests help doctors to determine if the cancer has spread. Individual patients may undergo different tests. However, all of these tests serve to help doctors determine the stage of cancer that a woman has. The system of staging widely used to describe cervical cancer is FIGO, which stands for International Federation of Gynecology and Obstetrics. FIGO classifies cervical cancer in stages 0 through IV.

STAGE 0 CERVICAL CANCER

If abnormal cervical cells are left untreated, then they will eventually develop into stage 0 cervical cancer. Stage 0 cervical cancer is also known as cervical carcinoma in situ. This is an early form of cervical cancer. At this stage, only the top layer of cervical cells is affected. The lesion,

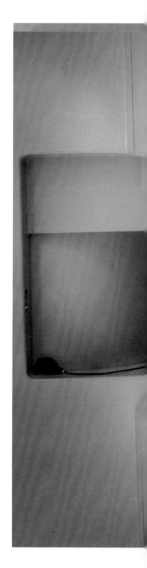

In this photograph, a patient is about to undergo an MRI test. Among many other uses, MRIs can be used to help a doctor to determine the stage of a woman's cervical cancer.

or area of abnormal tissue, is flat. Deeper layers of cervical tissue are not involved, and the cancer has not yet invaded nearby tissue. (The term *in situ* makes sense, then, as it is Latin for "in its place.") This stage of cancer may also be called noninvasive carcinoma. When explaining

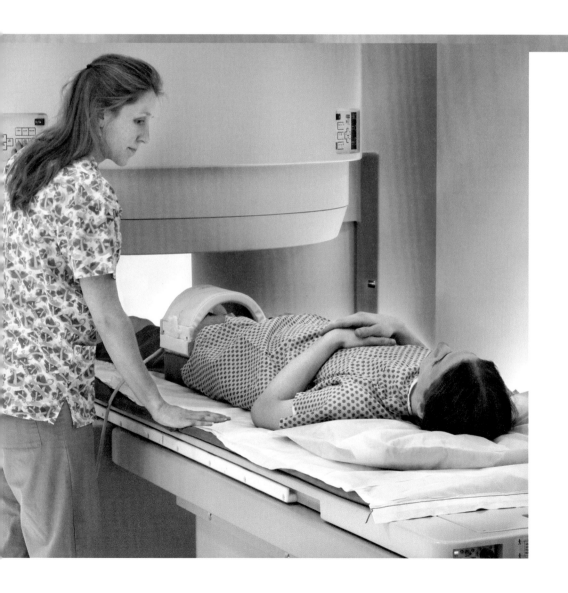

cervical cancer at this stage, most doctors will describe it as precancer. However, if left untreated, carcinoma in situ will develop into invasive cervical cancer. This is when the cancer begins to spread. Therefore, doctors will usually recommend that a stage 0 lesion be completely removed.

STAGE I CERVICAL CANCER

Stage I cervical cancer has not yet spread from the cervix. About 60 percent of women are in stage I

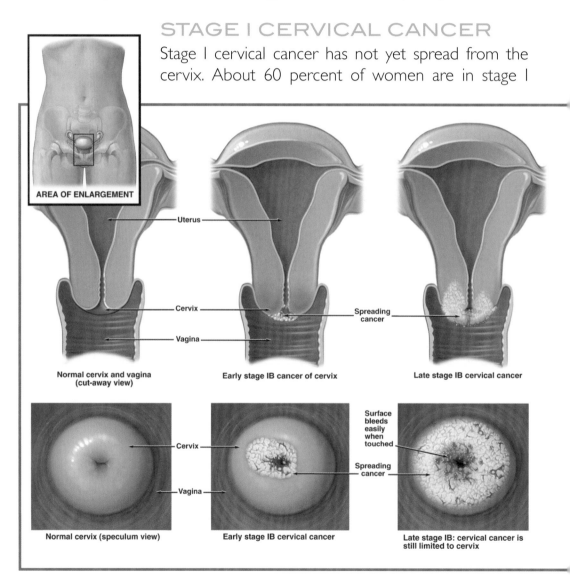

AREA OF ENLARGEMENT

Uterus

Cervix

Vagina

Normal cervix and vagina
(cut-away view)

Spreading cancer

Early stage IB cancer of cervix

Late stage IB cervical cancer

Cervix

Vagina

Normal cervix (speculum view)

Early stage IB cervical cancer

Surface bleeds easily when touched

Spreading cancer

Late stage IB: cervical cancer is still limited to cervix

when their cancer is discovered. This stage is divided into stages IA and IB, based on how much cancer is present. In stage IA, there is just a small amount of cancer, and it can only be seen with a microscope. The area of invasion is less than about 0.125 inch (5 millimeters) deep and less than about 0.25 inch (7 mm) wide. More than 95 percent of the women treated at this stage survive at least five years after treatment. In stage IB, there is more cancer present than in stage IA. In stage IB, the cancer can usually be seen without a microscope. The cancer may be larger than about 1.6 inches (4 cm). However, this stage also includes cervical cancers that can only be seen with a microscope but have spread deeper than about 0.20 inch (5 mm) into the cervical tissue or are wider than 0.25 inch (7 mm). Between 80 and 90 percent of the women treated at this stage survive at least five years after treatment.

STAGE II CERVICAL CANCER

In stage II cervical cancer, the cancer has spread beyond the cervix.

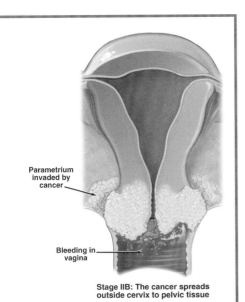

Parametrium invaded by cancer

Bleeding in vagina

Stage IIB: The cancer spreads outside cervix to pelvic tissue

Stage IIB cervical cancer

The illustrations at left show two different views of the progression of cervical cancer from normal (far left) to stage IIB cervical cancer (far right).

However, the cancer remains confined to the pelvic area. The pelvic area is located in the lower part of the abdomen between the two hip bones. Twenty-five percent of women are diagnosed with cervical cancer while it is in this stage. Stage II is separated into stages IIA and IIB, depending on where the cancer has spread. In stage IIA, the cancer has reached the upper two-thirds of the vagina. It has not spread as far as the lower third of the vagina. In stage IIB, the cancer has spread to the tissue next to the cervix. This tissue is called parametrial tissue. Sixty-five to 69 percent of women who are diagnosed with stage II cervical cancer survive for five or more years after receiving treatment.

STAGE III CERVICAL CANCER

Stage III describes cervical cancer that has spread to the lower part of the vagina or the pelvic wall. Only 10 percent of women are in stage III when their cervical cancer is discovered. At this stage, the cancer may be blocking the ureters, which are the tubes that carry urine from the

FIGURING OUT THE CAUSE OF CERVICAL CANCER

In the early 1900s, scientists discovered that cervical cancer was common in female sex workers (prostitutes) and was rare in nuns, except for those who were sexually active before they joined the convent. It was also noticed that cervical cancer was more common in women whose husbands had lost their first wives to cervical cancer. This led to the idea that cervical cancer could be linked to sexually transmitted disease. However, it was not until the 1980s that the human papillomavirus was identified as the main cause of cervical cancer.

kidneys to the bladder. The kidneys are located in the abdomen, or belly. They keep the fluids in the body balanced. The kidneys send extra fluid and waste to the bladder as urine. The bladder is then emptied when a woman goes to the bathroom.

Stage III cancer is divided into stage IIIA and stage IIIB. In stage IIIA, the cancer has spread to the lower third of the vagina, but it has not yet reached the pelvic wall. In stage IIIB cervical cancer, the cancer has reached the pelvic wall and may be blocking urine flow to the bladder. This may cause the kidneys to enlarge and stop working. According to another staging system by the American Joint Committee on Cancer, the cancer may also reach the lymph nodes in the pelvis during this stage. The lymph nodes are found in various places throughout the body. They are important in the body's fight against infection. Only about half of the women who are diagnosed with stage III cervical cancer (about 47 to 50 percent) live for five or more years after treatment.

STAGE IV CERVICAL CANCER

Stage IV is the last stage of cervical cancer. Only 5 percent of women are in this stage when their cervical cancer is first discovered. In stage IV, the cancer has left the pelvic region and has spread to nearby or more distant organs. Stage IV is separated into stages IVA and IVB, according to how far from the cervix the cancer has spread. In stage IVA, the cancer has spread to organs that are close to the cervix. These organs include the bladder, the kidneys, and the rectum. The rectum is the lower part of the large intestine. The large intestine functions to remove water from the digestive tract and form feces. In stage IVB, the cancer has spread to distant organs, farther from the cervix. These organs may include the lungs, stomach, and liver. At this stage, the patient's organs may not function normally. The patient may also experience severe pain. Only about 20 to 30 percent of women who are diagnosed with stage IV cervical cancer will live five years after treatment.

TEN GREAT QUESTIONS TO ASK YOUR DOCTOR OR GYNECOLOGIST

1. How often should I go to the gynecologist?

2. Am I too young to get a Pap smear?

3. What should I do if I have any itching, bleeding, or pain following a gynecologist exam?

4. What can I do to avoid getting the human papillomavirus?

5. Would you recommend I get the HPV vaccine?

6. What are the common side effects of the HPV vaccination?

7. What should I do if I am infected with HPV?

8. Does having HPV make me more vulnerable to other sexually transmitted diseases?

9. My mother (sister/grandmother/aunt) is infected with one of the HPV viruses that causes cervical cancer. Does this mean I am more likely to be infected with the same strain of HPV?

10. If I get cervical cancer, does it mean I won't be able to have children?

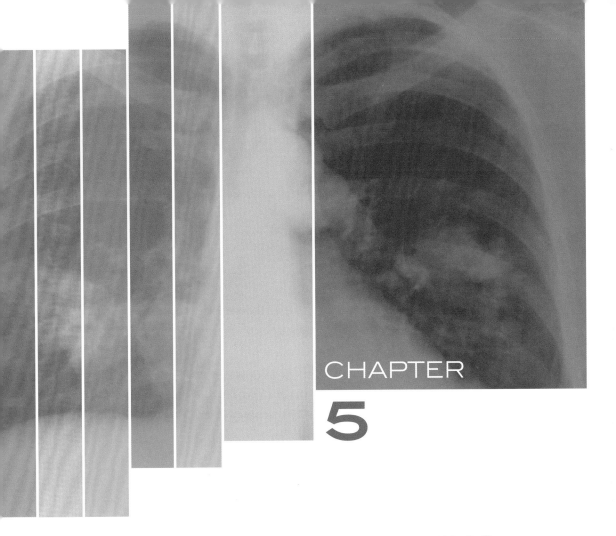

CHAPTER

5

TREATING AND PREVENTING CERVICAL CANCER

Survival rates for the different stages of cervical cancer are averages based on a large number of women. Nobody can predict with certainty what will happen to a cervical cancer patient, as each woman responds differently to treatment.

It is important to catch cervical cancer early, for survival rates fall as the cancer progresses. Therefore, it is wise to visit the gynecologist regularly. Once a doctor can determine what stage of cervical cancer a woman is in, a treatment plan can be made. Every stage of cervical cancer is treated differently. Depending on what stage the cancer is in, some treatment options include minor to major surgery, chemotherapy, and radiation.

TREATMENT OF PRECANCEROUS CELLS AND CARCINOMA IN SITU

Precancerous or abnormal cells are usually discovered in a Pap smear and are confirmed by a biopsy. Though this stage is not life threatening, it could become life threatening if nothing is done. A doctor may recommend one of several options. Loop electrosurgical extension procedure (LEEP), conization, and cryotherapy are the most common options. These procedures can also be used to treat cervical carcinoma in situ, or stage 0 cervical cancer. LEEP is the most popular treatment for a precancerous condition and is usually the first choice of treatment. This procedure can be carried out in the gynecologist's office. The abnormal cervical tissue is removed with a sharp wire loop. An electric current is passed through the loop, making it very hot. This allows the loop to easily slice through the cervical tissue. It also cauterizes (burns) the tissue as it goes, helping to stop the bleeding and serving to eliminate any remaining abnormal tissue. The process only takes about five minutes. This procedure is painless, but some women do experience cramping afterward. It takes three to six weeks for the cervix to heal.

Conization, or cone biopsy, removes more tissue than a regular biopsy. A surgical scalpel removes a cone-shaped section of cervical tissue. This procedure is usually done in a hospital, and the patient can go home that same day. Vaginal bleeding is normal for about one week after the procedure. Full healing takes about four to six weeks.

Cryotherapy involves freezing the abnormal cervical cells in order to kill them. A chemical, usually liquid nitrogen, is used to super-cool a metal probe. The probe is then held against the suspicious tissue. This freezes the abnormal cells. The damaged cells are then shed over the next few weeks as a clear discharge. This procedure can be done in

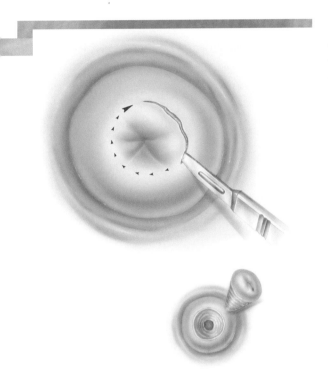

The illustration at left shows a cone-shaped section of the cervix being removed with a scalpel. This type of biopsy is called conization, or cone biopsy.

the gynecologist's office. During cryotherapy, most women experience cramp-like pain. It takes about three to six weeks to heal after the procedure. Following LEEP, conization, and cryotherapy, Pap smears should be done every three months for one year. This will help to ensure that all of the abnormal cells were removed.

SURGERY

Surgery is used to remove cancerous tissue from in or around the cervix. The deeper the cancerous cells have invaded the healthy tissue, the more tissue will have to be removed. In some cases, cervical cancer can be treated with a hysterectomy. This is the removal of the uterus and the cervix. Stage 0 and stage IA tumors can sometimes be treated in this way. Sometimes with a hysterectomy, the ovaries are removed as well. The ovaries produce female hormones such as estrogen. When the ovaries are removed, a woman will undergo menopause. Normal menopause, which marks the end of menstruation, usually occurs in women around the age of fifty. Other symptoms of menopause are vaginal dryness, hot flashes, and night sweats. Depending on her age and health, a woman having her ovaries removed might require hormone replacement therapy. This involves giving a woman a series of drugs to replace the hormones that her body is no longer able to make. These hormones can be delivered to the body in a number of ways, including patches, creams, pills, gels, and injections. A woman who is experiencing surgical menopause may undergo hormone replacement therapy until she reaches the age of natural menopause.

The ovaries also produce eggs. Though a woman undergoing a hysterectomy would not be able to carry a child, it is sometimes possible to remove some of her eggs and preserve them before the surgery. That way, she may be able to have a child later through the use of a surrogate mother. The eggs would be fertilized and placed into the uterus of the surrogate mother. The surrogate mother would then carry and give birth to the baby. When cervical cancer has invaded the tissue surrounding the cervix, a procedure called a radical hysterectomy may be performed. This surgery removes the cervix and the uterus, as well as tissue from the vagina and the lymph nodes in the pelvic region. Radical hysterectomies are performed for stages IA, IB, and IIA cervical cancers. A hysterectomy is major surgery. It is performed in a hospital. The physical recovery from a hysterectomy takes about four to six weeks. However, a lot of women are emotionally devastated by the loss of their reproductive organs. There are support groups to help these women.

RADIATION THERAPY

Radiation therapy uses high-energy radiation to kill cervical cancer cells. The radiation damages the DNA in the cells, causing them to die.

Cancer cells are more likely to be affected by the radiation because they divide more rapidly. However, some healthy cells are also destroyed during radiation therapy.

There are two types of radiation therapy: internal radiation therapy and external radiation therapy. With internal radiation therapy, a small capsule of radioactive material is placed directly in the cervix. This requires the patient to stay in the hospital for several days. The capsule is removed before the patient leaves the hospital. For early stages of cervical cancer, radiation therapy is an alternative to surgery. Stages 0

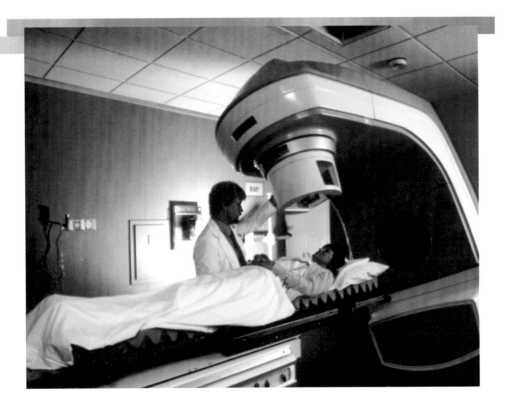

Above, a woman is about to undergo external radiation therapy. The machine being used is a linear accelerator, which emits a focused, high-voltage X-ray.

and IA cervical cancers are sometimes treated using internal radiation therapy. With external radiation therapy, a large machine points a beam of radiation at the patient's pelvic region. This type of radiation treatment does not require a hospital stay. The patient goes to the hospital to receive treatment when necessary but can go home that same day. Usually, a patient goes for treatment five days in a row for about six to eight weeks. External radiation therapy is usually used to treat more advanced stages of cervical cancer.

Radiation therapy is painless, but the trauma of irradiation can irritate cells, leading to negative side effects in the patient. The most common of these are tiredness, nausea, and loss of appetite. Radiation of the cervix can also destroy the ovaries, bringing on menopause. When radiation therapy is used to treat later stages of cervical cancer, it is used in conjunction with chemotherapy.

CHEMOTHERAPY

Chemotherapy, often referred to as just "chemo," is a type of treatment that uses chemicals or drugs to kill cancer cells. The two most common drugs used for the treatment of cervical cancer are cisplatin and 5-fluorouracil. These drugs keep cells from dividing. Most chemotherapeutic drugs are administered through an IV. The drugs enter the bloodstream and flow throughout the entire body. Therefore, chemotherapy is useful when the cervical cancer has spread to other parts of the body. Chemotherapy is used to treat stages IB, IIA, IIB, III, IVA, and IVB.

By itself, chemotherapy does not work that well for the treatment of cervical cancer. Therefore, it is given with radiation therapy. Combining radiation therapy with chemotherapy is much more effective against cervical cancer. Chemotherapy affects cancer cells because they are dividing rapidly. However, it affects other rapidly dividing cells in the body as well. Hair follicles, reproductive cells, and the cells lining the digestive

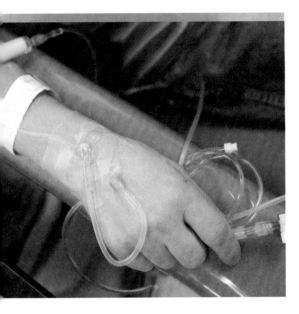

Tubes funnel chemotherapy drugs into a patient's body. The two most common chemotherapy drugs used for the treatment of cervical cancer are cisplatin and 5-fluorouracil.

tract all divide rapidly. Therefore, these cells, too, are affected by chemotherapy. This explains the hair loss, lowered fertility, and vomiting often associated with chemotherapy.

ADVANCES IN THE SCREENING AND PREVENTION OF CERVICAL CANCER

A new computerized instrument called the AutoPap makes the Pap smear easier and more accurate. Instead of having people read the Pap smear slides, the AutoPap reads them. However, a cytopathologist is still needed to review the slides that the AutoPap reads as abnormal. Sometimes, the AutoPap is used to reread slides that people have identified as normal. In many cases, it has identified abnormal cells that the humans missed.

The Polarprobe represents another advance in cervical cancer screening, although Polarprobe technology is still being developed and is, therefore, not yet ready for use. This portable device scans the cervix

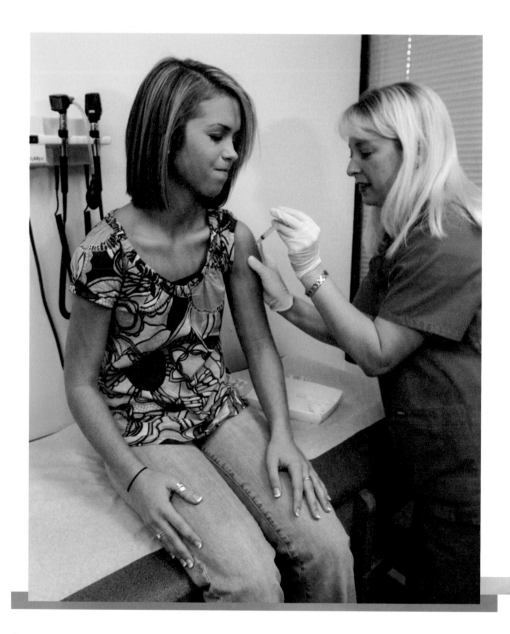

A nurse injects an eighteen-year-old patient with a shot containing the HPV vaccine. Many believe that this vaccine will reduce the number of cases of cervical cancer.

for cell changes. It does not scrape cells from the cervix, as is done with the Pap smear. Instead, the pen-shaped Polarprobe is inserted into the vagina and is simply passed over the cervix. The Polarprobe uses electrical and light pulses to identify normal and abnormal cells. The results would be ready by the end of the exam.

An advance in the prevention of cervical cancer is the development of the HPV vaccine. Vaccines help the body to fight off illnesses. They help the body to create antibodies. Antibodies are the body's defensive cells that fight off germs. The HPV vaccine contains virus-like particles (VLPs). To the body's immune system, these VLPs look like the real

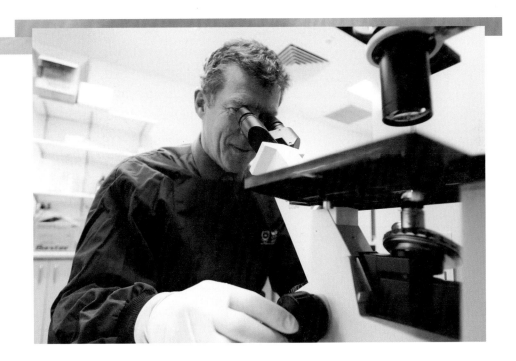

Professor Ian Frazer (above) developed a cervical cancer vaccine that protects women against the human papillomavirus. Cervical cancer is one of the few human cancers known to be directly caused by a virus.

HPV VACCINE DEATHS

The Food and Drug Administration (FDA) lists nausea, dizziness, pain, and itching as possible side effects of the HPV vaccination. The FDA claims that Gardasil, the HPV vaccine created by Merck, is safe. However, some do not agree. According to FoxNews.com in 2007, there have been more than three thousand adverse reactions to the vaccine. These include eight deaths in girls as young as nine years old. The National Vaccine Information Center (NVIC) is an organization that is dedicated to preventing childhood injury

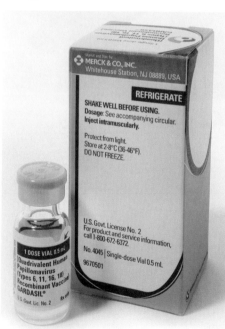

and death from vaccine. It has found reports listing seizures, joint pain, slurred speech, temporary loss of vision, severe headaches, and paralysis due to the Gardasil vaccine. The reactions listed have not been conclusively linked to Gardasil, however. The FDA and the Centers for Disease Control and Prevention believe there is no reason to reexamine the drug. Merck still recommends use of the vaccine.

Gardasil was approved by the Food and Drug Administration in June 2006. The drug is manufactured by Merck & Co., a pharmaceutical company.

human papillomavirus. However, the VLPs cannot actually cause the disease. When a woman is given the HPV vaccine, her body is tricked into making antibodies against the virus. Then, when she actually comes into contact with the virus, her body will be ready to fight it off.

Two pharmaceutical companies have HPV vaccines. GlaxoSmithKline developed Cervarix, which it claims protects against two different

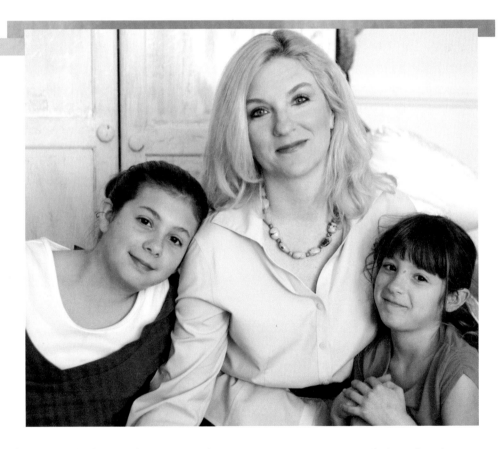

Cheryl Lieck (center), a cervical cancer survivor, poses with her daughters. Lieck supported legislation in Texas that would require sixth-grade girls to be vaccinated against HPV.

strains of cervical cancer–causing HPV. The other company, Merck, created a vaccine it calls Gardasil. It protects against the same two strains of HPV as Cervarix does. However, it also protects against two wart-causing strains of HPV. Gardasil has been available to the public since 2006. Cervarix was expected to become available in the United States in 2008. Gardasil is for use in females from ages nine to twenty-six.

A GOOD REASON FOR OPTIMISM

A discussion of cervical cancer should end on a good note. Techniques in the area of detection and diagnosis, which began with the Pap smear, continue to advance. Thanks to better technology, precancerous and cancer cells can be detected early. The number of women who die from cervical cancer has been greatly reduced because of new technologies, and it should continue to decline in the future.

Unlike Evita Perón, women today do not have to remain in the dark about their disease. The key is education and regular visits to the gynecologist. When cervical cancer is caught early, a woman has every reason to expect a complete recovery.

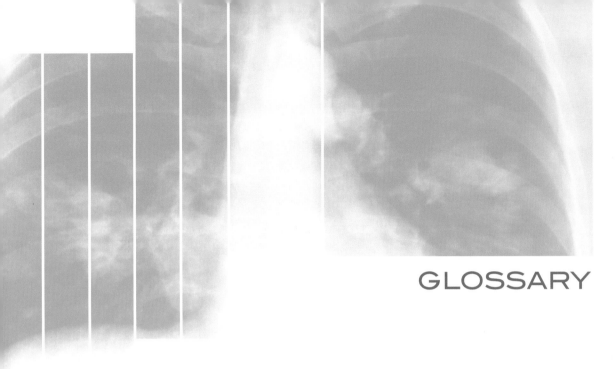

antibiotic Substance that is able to kill bacteria.

autoimmune deficiency syndrome (AIDS) Immune system disease caused by infection with human immunodeficiency virus (HIV).

biopsy Removal of a sample of tissue for laboratory tests.

bloodstream Flow of blood throughout the body.

cancer Illness caused by a tumor that destroys healthy tissue.

cell Basic unit of living things.

cell division Process by which a cell divides to form two new cells.

deoxyribonucleic acid (DNA) Substance that carries an organism's genetic information.

human immunodeficiency virus (HIV) Virus that causes AIDS.

immune system System of the body that recognizes and fights disease.

invasive cancer Cancer that tends to spread from one place to another in the body.

malignant Describing a cancer that is likely to grow or spread.

menopause Time in an older woman's life when her menstruation naturally stops.

menstruation Monthly discharge of blood and other matter from the uterus of a female that occurs between puberty and menopause.

metastasis Spread of a tumor from one part of the body to other parts of the body.

organ Independent part of the body that serves a specific function.

Pap smear Test to detect cancerous or precancerous cells in the cervix.

polyp A growth emerging from a mucous membrane.

radiation Energy emitted in the form of waves.

ribonucleic acid (RNA) Acid responsible for making protein.

tissue Group of similar cells in an organism.

tumor Abnormal mass of tissue.

virus Nonliving particle that consists of genetic material inside a protein capsule.

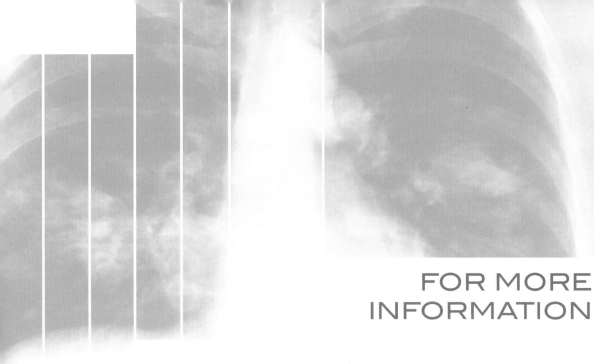

FOR MORE INFORMATION

American Social Health Association
P.O. Box 13827
Research Triangle Park, NC 27709
(919) 361-8400
Web site: http://www.ashastd.org
The American Social Health Association is a nonprofit organization
   dedicated to improving the health of people. Its main focus is
   preventing sexually transmitted diseases.

Centers for Disease Control and Prevention
1600 Clifton Road
Atlanta, GA 30333
(800) 311-3435
Web site: http://www.cdc.gov
The CDC is a major component of the U.S. Department of Health
   and Human Services. It promotes the health and quality of life of
   people by controlling disease, disability, and injury.

International Federation of Gynecology and Obstetrics
10 Theed Street
London SE 1 8ST
United Kingdom
+44 20 7928 1166
Web site: http://www.figo.org/index.asp
The FIGO is a worldwide organization that promotes the well-being
of women by raising the standards of practice in obstetrics and
gynecology.

National Cancer Institute
6116 Executive Boulevard, Room 3036A
Bethesda, MD 20892
(800) 4-CANCER (422-6237)
Web site: http://www.cancer.gov
The National Cancer Institute is a component of the U.S. National
Institutes of Health. It is dedicated to the prevention, diagnosis,
and treatment of cancer.

National Vaccine Information Center
204 Mill Street, Suite B1
Vienna, VA 22180
(703) 938-0342
Web site: http://nvic.org
The NVIC is an organization that works to prevent childhood injury
and deaths from vaccines.

National Women's Health Network
514 10th Street NW, Suite 400
Washington, DC 20004
(202) 628-7814

Web site: http://www.nwhn.org
The National Women's Health Network is a voice for all types of
women's health issues. Part of its mission is to advocate for women
in all aspects of their reproductive and sexual health.

WEB SITES

Due to the changing nature of Internet links, Rosen Publishing has
developed an online list of Web sites related to the subject of this book.
This site is updated regularly. Please use this link to access the list:

http://www.rosenlinks.com/cms/cerv

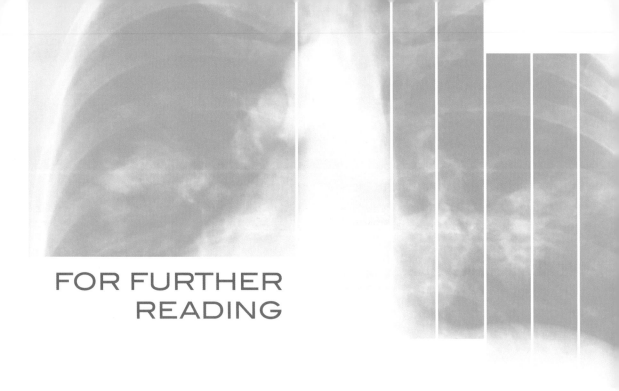

FOR FURTHER READING

Ayer, Pamela. *Crying in the Shower–Cervical Cancer*. Frederick, MD: PublishAmerica, 2005.

Carter, Elizabeth. *Everything You Need to Know About Human Papillomavirus*. New York, NY: Rosen Publishing Group, 2001.

Icon Health Publications. *Human Papilloma Virus–A Medical Dictionary, Bibliography, and Annotated Research Guide to Internet References*. San Diego, CA: Icon Health Publications, 2004.

Icon Health Publications. *The Official Patient's Sourcebook on Cervical Cancer: A Revised and Updated Directory for the Internet Age*. San Diego, CA: Icon Health Publications, 2002.

Nardo, Don. *Human Papillomavirus (HPV) (Diseases and Disorders)*. Farmington Hills, MI: Lucent Books, 2007.

Shoquist, Jennifer, and Diane Stafford. *The Encyclopedia of Sexually Transmitted Diseases* (Library of Health and Living). New York, NY: Facts on File, 2004.

Spencer, Juliet. *Cervical Cancer* (Deadly Diseases and Epidemics). New York, NY: Chelsea House Publications, 2007.

Stanley, Deborah. *Sexual Health Information for Teens: Health Tips About Sexual Development, Human Reproduction, and Sexually Transmitted Diseases* (Teen Health Series). Detroit, MI: Omnigraphics, 2003.

Szarewski, Anne. *Preventing Cervical Cancer: What Every Woman Should Know*. St. Albans, UK: Altman Publishing, 2007.

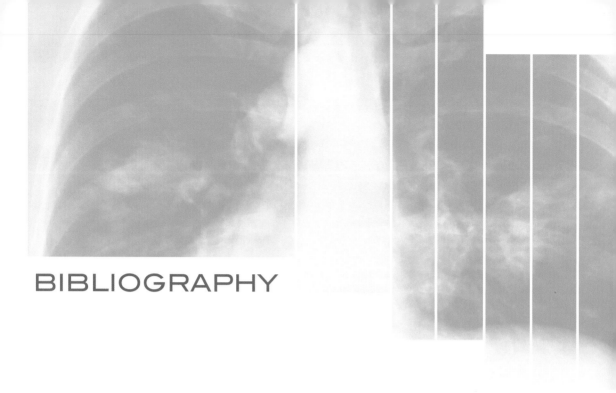

BIBLIOGRAPHY

Benowitz, Steven I. *Cancer.* Berkeley Heights, NJ: Enslow Publishers, 1999.

Fred Hutchinson Cancer Research Center. "Cervical Cancer." 2008. Retrieved March 11, 2008 (http://www.fhcrc.org/research/diseases/cervical_cancer).

The Health Resource Incorporated. "Cervical Cancer." Retrieved March 11, 2008 (http://www.thehealthresource.com/cancer_info/cervical_cancer3.cfm).

Ingraham, J. L., and C. A. Ingraham. *Introduction to Microbiology.* 3rd ed. Pacific Grove, CA: Brooks/Cole-Thomson Learning, Inc., 2004.

National Cancer Institute. "Cancer Reference Information." Revised March 26, 2008. Retrieved March 11, 2008 (http://www.cancer.org/docroot/CRI/content/CRI_2_4_1X_What_is_cervical_cancer_8.asp).

Raasch, Marsha. "Questions About Gardasil: Cervical Cancer Vaccine and Your Daughter." *Associated Content*, February 21, 2007. Retrieved March 11, 2008 (http://www.associatedcontent.com/article/149745/questions_about_gardasil_cervical_cancer.html).

Runowicz, Carolyn D., M.D., Jeanne A. Petrek, M.D., and Ted S. Gansler, M.D. *Women and Cancer: A Thorough and Compassionate Resource for Patients and Their Families.* New York, NY: Villard Books, 1999.

Spencer, Juliet V. *Cervical Cancer.* New York, NY: Chelsea House Publishers, 2007.

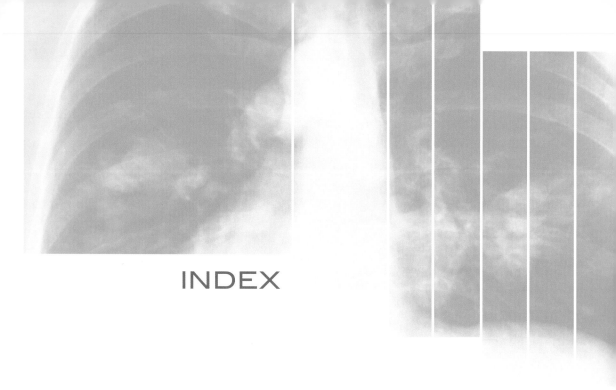

INDEX

ABOUT THE AUTHOR

Heather Hasan graduated from college summa cum laude with dual majors in chemistry and biochemistry. She has written many young adult books about science and has authored books on the subjects of astronomy and genetics. She currently lives in Pennsylvania with her husband, Omar, and their sons, Samuel and Matthew.

PHOTO CREDITS

Cover, p. 1 © Steve Gschmeissner/Photo Researchers; cover (corner photo), pp. 4, 5 © Punchstock; back cover National Cancer Institute; p. 5 Keystone/Hulton Archive/Getty Images; p. 10 adapted from © www.istockphoto.com/Thomas Paschke; p. 12 Joanna Cameron © Dorling Kindersley; p. 14 © Biophoto Associates/Photo Researchers, Inc.; pp. 16, 30 World Health Organization publication, *Comprehensive Cervical Cancer Control: A Guide to Essential Practice*; p. 19 © Kwangshin Kim/Photo Researchers, Inc.; p. 21 Shutterstock.com; p. 23 Pascal Le Segretain/Getty Images; p. 27 © Mark Thomas/Photo Researchers, Inc.; p. 29 Walter Sanders/Time & Life Pictures/Getty Images; pp. 34–35 Lester Lefkowitz/Photographer's Choice/Getty Images; pp. 36–37 nucillustration/Newscom; p. 43 pttmedical/Newscom; p. 45 © Larry Mulvehill/Photo Researchers, Inc.; p. 47 Chris Hondros/Getty Images; pp. 48, 51© AP Images; p. 49 Jonathan Wood/Getty Images; p. 50 Russell Kirk/Merck & Co. via Getty Images.

Designer: Evelyn Horovicz; Editor: Christopher Roberts;
Photo Researcher: Cindy Reiman